WHEN I BLEED

When I Bleed

Poems about Endometriosis

MAGGIE BOWYER

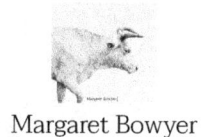

Margaret Bowyer

Thank you to those who believed my pain
and always support me.
Thank you to all of the strong and lovely
warriors who helped me get here.

Maggie Bowyer
Greensboro, North Carolina
www.maggiebowyer.com
hello@maggiewrites.com

IBSN: 9780578867878
LCCN:
Printed in the United States of America
First Printing, 2021

Endometriosis

You took my life
And my liberty;
Happiness ran towards
The sunset
So long ago
I still question
If I ever met this
Mysterious emotion.
Tell me this:
Where can I go now
To seek justice?
Will I ever find
Freedom?

2020

One might want to read
Happy words;
That's not what
You'll find here.
Here is where I bleed,
Where I stitch myself
Back together,
Piece by piece.
You want an outpouring
Of something joyous,
But all the laughter
Has been compressed out of me
After a year this heavy.
I do not have
Rivers of rhyme
Or oceans of odes;
I only have tears.
We can sit
On wooden floorboards
And share the somber silence
Of the night, if you'd like.

We Were So Close

You slipped rejection
Underneath my tongue
Like a slow-acting poison;
It has taken years
To finish the old me off.

I want to write new poems
About fresh ideas
But nothing will come out.
As though once I released
All my trauma on the page,
The cat got my tongue
And killed my creativity.
It's like once I was done healing
I ceased to be.

The burns didn't hurt this badly
When we were on fire.

- Disassociation

I wanted to be
A flying corpse.
Swinging high above the grass,
I imagined flinging myself
From the swing set.
I swore then that
My shoulders
Unhinged from my arms,
My torso found its home
In mid-air
And I was soaring.

– and then it flipped

Would I recognize you
If we passed on the street?
Were we connected
By anything but
An umbilical cord
And your need for control?
If we met now,
If we met differently,
Do you think
You would've learned
From me?

- Mother knows best

Dirty Girls' Disease

They told me
I was sick
Because I let you
Find a home
Deep inside me.

They told me
I must be dirty,
Sex with demons,
Sip this clean juice,
Have you tried yoga?

Is this pain
Ripping me -
Ripping us -
Apart, really just
Psychosomatic?

There are bolts
Where my hips
Should be.
Loosening,
They pinch me.
Tightening,
They strip me
To the core.

I still want to yell
About all of the hell
You raised right through me.

-I'm too tired

There are countless days
When I wish I could
Pack up my heart
And run away,
Leave my body behind.
I want to ride the rails
Of the universe's light trails,
Escape into the unknown
Rather than be stuck
In this immobile rutt.

I want to find my soul
Rather than lose it.

PTSD Does Funny Things

Sometimes when I am
Speeding down the highway,
I envision the wheels of my car
Flying off in every direction;
70 miles an hour,
Wind and snapping metal
Fills our ears
Above the shrieking bass.
If I dote on this daydream
I'll stall out
Freak out
Jerk the car from left to right
Trying to stabilize.
The picture is fleeting,
Traveling just as fast
Through my memories.

I was only ten
The first time I remember
Getting stabbed.
My agony pierced the air
With a sickening scream.

My mom barreled down the hall,
Just as the knife seemed to vanish.
Minutes into me explaining
This random phantom pain,
It struck, so suddenly,
Same as before.
My shriek struck her face
Before either of us realized
I was crumbling to the floor.

Only a decade on this earth
And I felt at death's door;
Worried faces rushing
Me into emergency rooms
Where there is endless waiting;
Nothing seems remotely urgent
To the late-night workers.
The nurse made me drink
Medicine colored lavender,
Smelling of paste;

I've never liked the taste
Of a hospital stay.
They didn't find appendicitis,
Smiled,
And sent me on my way.

I woke up to sheets soaked in blood.
Months and months,
Years and years;
No one told me
Your body should not be
Maimed by your monthly.

I Hate it Here

I don't think you can understand
How it feels to be this hollow,
Like every bone in your body
Is borrowed,
Struggling to survive
Off of minutes on loan,
Loaded with interest.

I used to think
These friends were mine.
How quick it switches
From laughing on armrests
And making this a place
We can all rest
To darkened looks in corridors,
Accentuated by whispers -
Apparently, I am a liar.
How does it all tumble down
Faster than a broken elevator
As it rushes to kiss
The floor of the basement?
Did you focus on my words
And not hers?
Did you see the way she chased me
Down the hall in a rage,
As I tried to make my escape?
Do you remember
The friendship we shared
Before all of the mess
Of falling in love?
How can you blame me
For these window shattering sobs
When she left me with a simple
"I need to get my heart broken

By someone else."
Did you forget the days before
She started getting leads?
Or is that why
You're still riding her coattails?
Why you followed her
All the way to LA?
Is that apartment I called home
Now a frozen tomb
Filled and sealed with
All our memories
Still sitting on the kitchen bar?
Did we forget to save
The daisies trying
To push their way up
In our rush to leave behind
The spider webs and regrets?
Is there a way to thaw this,
Work it out?
It's going to snow again
Later this week;
I wonder if I called you,
Would you be able to trade
The armor and daggers
For snowflakes on tastebuds?
To make snow angels,
Like the first few years
We celebrated finishing finals?
Would this blanket of white
Put our differences to bed?
Or will it at least leave me
With the silence I crave
To help me forget the way
You would sing in the candlelight

When the power went out?
Has this flicker of friendship finally
Succumbed to the falling snow?
I guess if you never read this,
I will never know.

(G)ee

(I) feel like shit.

(Physical) Therapy

My body started training
For a marathon
10 years ago,
And quite literally
Hasn't stopped running since.
Even running while I slept.
After physical therapy,
All I can muster
Are a few pets for my cats
As I collapse on the couch,
Unable to lift
My hands above my head
For the rest of the day.
Will every week
Go on this way?

Grief is in the questions
For which I have no answers,
In the hoops I am meant
To soar through just
To understand better
What my body is going through.
I curse the rain clouds
As I pound on my steering wheel
Screaming
"For the love of God
If you weren't going to be a parent,
There is no apparent reason
For my suffering!"
I might have wanted
A few more life lessons,
But the minimum courtesy
You could have given me
Was a conversation
About my impending
Disability.
Instead,
You left me,
Only to get sicker.
Only to end up like you.

Mutilation

Nails grip my scalp,
Rip hair right off
The back of my head.
I wish I could
Peel the skin away,
Tear through muscles
Until I find the neurons
That keep zapping me
With lightning bolts
To the stomach,
Metal stakes straight
Through my heel,
The aching fire in my arms
That engulfs my fingers
Before I can begin
The self lobotomy.

It is impossible
To recall
A time when
My body was
Not home
To this
Relentless
Pain.

I am a kitchen
Without plates,
Pots,
Pans.
I can burn
Pain into
My skin
On the burners;
I can gut myself
With utensils
That seem to serve
No other purpose.
What is the point
Of a kitchen
When my home
Has been destroyed?

What Was I Supposed to Do?

I was never supposed
To save you.
My only job
Was to be your child.

I cannot slice myself open
For you to believe me.
I cannot keep hiding
That this disability
Is breaking me, bone by bone.
I will not let myself
Disappear into the pain,
Disassociate to function.
What for?
A few more dollars
I'll see in my lifetime?
While the rich feast
On the working class's
Carnage,
We breathe in a virus.
For what?
Capitalist survival.

Invisible Demons

Can a branding
Cut so deep
It tears ligaments
At their seams,
Searing me
To my core?
As I writhe
In the bathtub,
Someone reaches up
From hell -
Or close enough -
Yanking my bones
With flaming hands,
My skin not showing
The torn
And burned
Edges of my nerves.

Clots

Grief
Is what I see
Starting back at me.
Pooled
In the toilet bowl
Are the most
Painful parts of me,
Passing.

I want to carve
My insides
Out
With a rusty spoon.
It would be
Far less painful.

I am in social
Isolation.
I'm not sure my body
Will give me any other
Option.

This part of me
Bumps and brushes
All the other
Parts of my identity.
I am so much more
Than the fire I stand in;
This inferno is not who I am,
But am I even recognizable
Under the third-degree burns
Smoking me from
The inside out?
This disease is
Impacting everything,
Even if it's not all of me.

I think I lost a part of myself.
It's often hard to tell,
When every cycle
Leads to heavy clots,
How can I know
If I lost a baby by now?

The Breakups We Don't Talk About

I miss you
Even more than I miss
The million little things
That have slipped through
The cracks in my body.
I miss drinking myself silly,
You trying to out drink me
And walking home petting
Every fire hydrant on the way.
Do you miss me, too?
I miss walking a few blocks
Just to dance my ass off;
The ability to drop everything
And rush over
In your free time.
I've lost so much time
Searching for a moment
I am free of this pain.
I miss you,
But more so
I miss who I could've been
If this disease wasn't wrecking me.
I miss myself
Far more than you could

Begin to understand;
I can promise this
As surely as I can promise
This friendship was broken by
Time and life changes
We cannot control.
I wish things could
Stay the same as 18 forever,
But my body is aging now
Faster than before;
I can't drink 40s
Like they're water
All summer.
Can you forgive me,
For abandoning you
When I lost myself?

Days like today
I am glad
For the emptiness
In my womb.
I couldn't bear
To pass down
Heirlooms as
Heinous
As this.
I am sorry,
To my unborn baby,
That we could
Never meet.
I promise,
It's less painful
This way.

My whole childhood
I believed your losses
Were my failures.
The real failure
Is a system
That let you get
So sick,
So sick of being sick,
That you dealt with it.
There's a sense of
Finality.
Control.
You finally garnered
Strength in your story.
Too bad
I had to lose (you)
For you to win.

Nothing but Pain

There is acid pouring
Through my abdomen,
Contained poorly
By barbed wires,
Cut only by the knife
Slicing through
My most tender points.

When we're in public
And the flare begins,
It registers as a simple
Contortion of expression
Or a hissing of my breath.
The grace of being home is
That I no longer have to waste
Energy on looking okay.
I fall to the ground
Screaming,
No one around
To hear me,
Thankfully.
I'd rather suffer in silence
Than be subjected
To deafening stares.
I feel like I'm in
An abusive relationship
With my body;
No one can see the bruises.

Casual Ableism

Shaking,
The familiar
Feeling washes
Over me;
It is not
A gentle rain.
It's not even
A torrential downpour
That leaves you
Clean.
No, it's actually
A shower with
Hard water hitting
My tender skin.
The heat turned up
As high as it goes,
Each time the water
Pounded with minerals
Beats my bare shoulders
It draws lines
Of pain
And grime
Along my skin.
This feeling is familiar.

Trying my hardest,
Scrubbing at this illness
As though the longer
I lingered,
Cleaning,
My pain would dissipate.
Don't they know
This disease
Doesn't work that way?
The harder I fight
Against my own body
And it's divine design,
The more I disappoint you
By not making 'progress.'
The more I push
To be able
The more my body rebels.
Don't they know
This disease
May always be this
Relentless?

Pain-somnia

The exhaustion rolls in
Like a storm over the ocean,
Black clouds tumbling
Over one another
In their race towards the shore.
At first, the clouds cried,
Sobbed into the ocean's abyss.
These storms quickly
Realized their pain fell
Onto deaf waves,
White noise of chronic pain,
And simply floated away;
This tempest refuses
To be tempered.
Instead, she cracks the sky
Wide-open with her
Screams of lightning strikes
And shakes the shore
With thunderous blows.
No matter my exhaustion
From trying to stay afloat,
I must keep swimming
Towards an invisible shore.

Grief wrapped in ribbon,
A presence taken
On your favorite holiday.
Now I'm left to
Dress it up in cheer
Even though its another year
You're not here.

It Just Takes Once

This isn't delicate.
It was never handled
As though it were
Specially marked 'fragile.'
This is a body.
A fighter.
An iron man.
Each time I fell,
I rose unscathed.
Even if I got
A chip or scratch
The king's men ran in,
Patched me together again;
Until I felt this body,
This human vessel,
Shatter
From being dropped
Too many times before.
There is no knight
Or surgeon alike
Who can fix this.

The real heartache
Comes in fleeting moments.

Your mom mentioning
Holding onto a baby book
For us one day.

A surrogacy subplot
Appearing out of the blue
On my new TV show.

My half birthday,
When I was officially older
Than my mom was
When she lost
Any future fruits
From her tree,
Finally uprooted.

Saying congratulations
And wanting to mean it,
So desperately
That I hate myself when
I disappear for the bathroom
During your sister's baby shower,
Only to have my own shower,

An outpouring of grief
For a happiness
I might never reach.

The mourning happens
In the middle of the night,
When I'm lying awake,
Still in pain,
Listening to you snore,
Alone with my thoughts.
In the thousands of moments
Of loss surrounding me,
I hold my face frozen,
Only thawing when
Everyone I love
Is fast asleep;
When no one can hear
How I hum for you in heaven.

-My stolen lullabies

You're Gone

Missing answers
To what-ifs
I shouldn't have
Bothered asking.

I Died Trying

Hour after hour,
Bite after bite
Taken out of my strength,
Trying to explain
That I can't lift a bowling ball
Or go out drinking,
But that I miss you
More than anything.
I can't keep reaching out
Through a video call
You forgot about.
You can't keep showing up
Three hours late;
By then, the fatigue
Is dictating my evening.
I do not need you
To get a medical degree,
Operate on me,
Or even understand.
But I can't keep
Giving away spoons
For people who
Never stay to eat.

This place still feels haunted,
But I'm getting good at
Ignoring ghouls and
Ghastly memories
When they jump out at me.

I'm Doing My Best

This is the most
I have ever loved myself,
And yet it is still
Far from enough.

Fatigue

Do you ever
Dust the table
With a tissue
Because you
Desperately
Want to clean
But your legs
Refuse to carry you,
And the side table
Is closer than the
Cleaning supplies
Neatly tucked away
Under the kitchen sink?

Pain Erases People

There are versions
Of myself
I will never recover,
Stolen by moments
I will forever remember.

Brain fog

I've misplaced:

My keys
     My wellness
          My heart
               My body
          My abilities
     My friendships
My life.

I found my keys
In the freezer.

I wonder if
I'll ever find
Myself.

Melancholia

Originally published in Written Tales

The chill creeps in
As I sit in the window.
Smoke puffs from
The chimney next door.
Ivy covered in frost
And icicles fall;
December sinks in
Like a cold-shouldered
Old friend.
I try to stretch,
Reach my toes,
But my own bones
Feel covered in snow.

Will You Be Waiting For Me?

Was God tired of
Watching Their child suffer?
Did They call you
Home gracefully?
Did your body decide
It was more drained
Than your palms,
Raised in praise?
Was there nothing left
To be thankful for?
Was the only thing
You could pray for
An end to the pain?
Did God walk you home
Peacefully,
Or did you fight valiantly
Against evil, to end up
Exhausted at heaven's gate?
Did God feel overcome
By Their remorse
That they forgave
Your final choice?

Spring

This world has grown
Far too warm
For our icicles
To remain beautiful.
All that's left
Is to see if they fall
Only to be shattered
On the slick asphalt,
Or slowly drip
Down tree branches,
Dragging out
Inevitable defeat.

I had to make my mind
A safe space to hide.
When my body
Tries to expel this disease
I feel the need to recede,
Step away from a being
That has become only pain.
I retreat into my own
Mental palace.
I fill my world with
Podcasts and internet friends,
Characters from
Books and shows;
They are always just
A few clicks away.
I can sit here numb,
For hours.
This is not depression.
Sometimes I wish it was,
Because maybe then
I would feel less guilty.
This comatose state
Is one of my choosing;
It is the best pain management
I can manage.

Good Timing

If you had met me
In high school
I would have eaten
Your heart, still warm.
You're far too kind,
And I was not kind enough
To myself.

An Apology to Myself

I am sorry
I didn't believe
In my own pain
Until I gathered
The courage
To share my life
Out loud.

Countless pelvic exams
Always lead me
To gulping down gasps
While my knuckles
Turn so white they
Bleed straight into
The crinkling paper
Plastered under my thighs.
Gloved fingers lead to
Trying to catch tears
In my eyelashes,
To halt hysteria
Lest this doctor, too,
Blame pelvic pain
On the brain.

-Pelvic pain shouldn't be normalized

Identity Crisis

I spent so much time
Attempting to be different
Than the woman
Who raised me;
I forgot to ask myself
Who I wanted to be.

Ambiguous loss is defined
As a loss that occurs
Without closure or understanding.

Ambiguous loss is defined
As all of their clothes returned to Carter's,
Quickly declining store credit or exchange.
All of these items bought in excitement
Returned with red-rimmed eyes,
Bags held in shaky hands -
Why won't the clerk stop staring?
They should understand.
Ambiguous loss is defined
As something no one can understand.
The ache of what could have been,
Hopes and dreams
Burned at the gravesite,
Wondering what my baby sister
Would have looked like,
What my little brother's
Laugh would have sounded like.
Ambiguous loss is not easily defined,
And less easily let go of.
How do you let go of the siblings
You never got to hold,
Got to know?

Someone once told me
It should be easier -
There are no memories to
Release like balloons,
No conflicts never to be resolved.
Ambiguous loss is defined
As the sibling rivalries
I would kill for,
They would have lived for.
It is defined as withholding hope
On a subsequent pregnancy
All the way through 37 weeks
Because if I grew to love the baby
As the woman's body grows to protect it,
I might not recover.
I often wonder what ambiguous loss
Is like for them -
Are Gus and Ellie waiting
Just outside the gates of heaven
For their mommy and daddy,
Brothers,
Me?
Are they just as lost and confused?
Do their bodies crave our hugs
As much as our arms ache
From reaching out?
Do they know their names,
Are they stuck in between,
Can they walk,
Can they fly,
Can they feel the love I have for them,
The pain I shed for them?
Is their loss just as ambiguous as mine?
Are they still waiting for this feeling

To be defined,
For closure so impossible to find?

Ambiguous loss is defined
As a loss that occurs
Without closure or understanding.
I understand that God needed
Two more angels,
But how am I supposed to close a book
When the first words were never written?

Reminders

If there were once
Good days
Then, logically,
There will be
Good days again.

I heat the teapot up
But the water is
Quickly filling me up.
I am sinking
To the kitchen floor.
Cried a river
That was too weak
To carry me to bed,
And so I will
Weep on the laminate
While the whistle
Rings in my fragile ears,
Lament for the energy
I have in fuzzy dreams,
No strength to stand for peppermint
To soothe my scratching throat
Or warm my frigid soul.

I feel like a stranger
Standing in my own skin.
Scars from surgeries
Wiped from my memory,
Parts taken out of me,
Pathologies that have
Changed everything
Yet nothing about me.

I lie atop
A mountain of shards.
Each bit of pain
Tries to dig in its fangs,
Cause me to crumble
Into a puddle of despair.

One day I will taste
Fresh air
Pass between these lips.
Someday I will be able
To stand again.

The bathroom linoleum
Cradles my hot skin.
This will pass,
I whisper to myself.
It always does.

When it finally dissipates,
I know I will stand up,
Straighten my shirt,
Try to pretend I still remember
My name or the date.

I will rise back up soon enough.
This body has been through
Far better and far worse.
This body has gotten me here.
This body has walked
On glass splinters for years
And I am still here.

Three Ways to Love Me

Let me fill my head
With maddening poetry, words
That distract me from the lyrics
Of our daily conversations.
Let me lay my head
In your lap and please,
Do not mock me for
Pinning my feet up
Against the wall and
Crushing a heating pad
Against my abdomen.
Please bring me weed,
Even when I don't ask for it;
I usually win the game
Of putting off medication
That would make it easier
To meditate despite the pain.
I forgo the little relief
A simple plant can bring.
I fear I am turning
Into a statue in the garden;
My mom must've become
Medusa;
I can barely move my legs,

My feet already turned to stone.
I know this paranoia
Would be exhaled
With a big cloud,
The fire in my legs
Would become embers
In my center;
These daggers in my abdomen
Turn to day-old surgery wounds;
I will be able
To actually talk to you.
I leave this note on your pillow,
On a Saturday morning.
While I sneak away
For my weekly appointment,
I hope you will learn
That I'm harder on myself
Than I ever mean to be
When it comes to you.
I know a simple apology
Won't always be enough so
Tell me, what can I do
To better love you?

Those aches and cramps
You're experiencing
Are valid and real.

I'm happy that you
Are planning your childbearing
By years and numbers.

Thank you for hiring me,
Taking a chance
In the midst of a pandemic.

I hold my tongue
A thousand different ways
Every single day.
I don't want to
Make this all about me,
But my heart is breaking
When every word you say
Penetrates my fragile senses.

-invisible illness

I'm Not Sure How I Feel Today

There are days
I am getting through it,
And days I am learning
To live with it.

I long ago
Let go
Of picturing love
And how we'd grow.
We water our thoughts
And mine are full
Of anxious weeds
Trying to take root in me.
I stopped staring at
The ground beneath my feet.
I let the skies
Fall onto my seeds
And grow what I need.
I'd much rather
Tend to you and me,
In the moment,
What we need.

Full Time

Originally published in A Cornered Gurl

I wonder if they called
The supermarket where I worked
Back in college, when
The thought of food
Sent me to the restroom
And some days my arms
Would suddenly give out
While I carried milk
Across the store floor.
I wonder if they heard
About the migraines
With quarter-sized blind spots.
I pray that they just saw
The impressive credentials,
The fact that I managed
To be a manager
From high school
Through college.
My paranoia tells me
They sense I hovered
On the page where I refused
To disclose my disability.
Did they know they were

Seated before someone
Who can slip off to puke
And return unaffected?
I've learned how to collapse
In that moment before fainting,
When your heart is racing
And the world zooms out
And the heat is turned up
And your hands are clammy
And you know to never reach out,
Expecting someone to catch you;
No, no instead you reach
Down and back --
I figured out quickly
How not to get a concussion
Every time my body and brain
Disconnect and I wake up
With lights spinning back
Into their bulbs above me.
They say it's frustrating
To employ someone who suddenly
Faints and can't come in
The next day,
Despite the fact I can still work
More effectively than anyone
When my pain is creeping
Above a level six.
Shouldn't it be considered
An asset to admit disability
On your resume?

No One Left to Blame

If I cut myself open
Would I bleed poetry?
If I could take
A scalpel
To the very spots
The doctors left scars,
Would it hurt less
Than their failures?
Would they finally
Become my failures?

Tiny little scars born of battles
Still being fought beneath them.
There is a part of me
That fears these walls
Are as far as my dreams go.
I am so frustrated
By a world that cannot see
That, given the chance,
My worst work
Would top their best.
I fear I will live in a world
That can not accommodate
Anyone who does not,
Cannot,
Will not,
Grind themselves until their
Bones begin to scream
Like a train warning:
Stop!
A crash is fast approaching.
I am exhausted
Because capitalism
Wasn't made for this body.

-I am sick enough; I cannot work myself to death

Rx: Research

Have I been buried alive
By chronic pain?
I can taste the dirt
As they put me in the earth,
Thick on my lips
Like the honey that drips
From doctor's lips.
Try this one,
They say.
There are no side effects,
They lie.
I swallow them whole.
When you're starved
For a moment of relief,
You'll eat their poison
By the mouth full,
No questions
Until the digestion
Leads to new problems.

It is strange
The snapshots of moments
I have collected
With the people
I have loved;
And there have been
A lot.

Each moment a kaleidoscope
Of polaroids and VHS clips,
Of safety nets and free falls,
Never quite the memory
I expect
When I go searching
For those I have loved.

-brainspotting

There are moments
I can't go back to,
Mistakes
I can't take back.
There are no more
Opportunities
For forgiveness
Unless it comes
From myself.

Always Waiting

Cancelation after cancelation,
There is no consolation
For the chronically ill.
To not only be trapped
In my own body,
But be at the mercy
Of schedulers and systems
That see us as dollar signs
And difficult drug seekers,
Is a perpetual
Predatory
Purgatory.

Appointment Armor

Some days there's
A fight in me.
There's a burning
Heap of flames
Where my body
Used to be.
Some days I am alight
With feverish frustration
That keeps me
Fighting for the
Hope of something
Ever getting better.
Today,
I need a nap
Before I don battle gear
To take a swing at
The medical system.

Endo Belly

I learned how to
Hate my body
Long before I desired
To love my body.
A preteen with
A bulging abdomen
Surrounded by judgment,
I learned to never
Give myself the breath
My lungs desperately craved,
Lest my core expand
Beyond my control.
There is a constant
Reframing process
Happening in my mind,
Even as I scan my body
For any looming threats.
We are at war;
I have to remind myself
We are on the same side.

When I hear the creak
Of the front door,
The jingle of keys,
I sigh, heavy but relieved.
When your grin strikes,
For a millisecond,
A finite moment,
I can forget.
I can take a deep breath
In this singular moment,
Open my diaphragm
And release my pelvic floor.

-Thank you for being my peace

There are versions of myself
I would have left,
And versions of myself
I would have kept.
The beauty in growing up
Is that you get to choose
Who you'll be tomorrow.

When the door closes
And clothes fall
From tired shoulders,
I assume I am alone.

The pain contorts
My fatigued face muscles;
Then I notice him,
Standing stone still in scrubs,
Sulking in the corner.
As I lie on the table,
The fear is familiar.

Though his hands
Are different,
And in different places,
Their weight on my ankles
Feels like shackles.
I glance at the door,
Latched tight.

Fingers grip my leg,
Tighter now as he tries
To extract vulgar phrases
From my frozen body.
As he begins

To stick needles in me,
Begging me to let
Dirt drip from my lips,
I felt no options
But to give in.

-Sexual violence isn't always a sexual act

No matter how many times
I have crumpled up,
Lied on the floor in vain attempts
To combat the waves of nausea
And blackout moments
Of blinding pain building,
I eventually rise again;
Every time.
This body is a miracle,
Pushing through pulsating,
Pounding pain
To survive every day.
This body is a divine being
That so bravely fights
The very thing nearly
Crippling me.

Tiny little scars.

Tiny little reminders.

Tiny little details in my story of

Survival.
Grief.
Pain.
Answers.
Agony.

My fingers will always
Find their place
At the base of your spine,
Trace up a line,
Remind you it's fine
To relax every once in a while.
The ghosts and ghouls
Can rest in the shadows,
We will deal with them tomorrow;
Right now let's sit down,
Watch as Christmas lights
Twinkle, light up your eyes
With a smile as wide as mine.
When you feel my
Fingernails trace your spine,
Reminding you of all the nights
We have spent together,
You can rest easy, finally
Knowing it will only get better.

This Isn't The End

The very act of
Surviving
In a world that does
Nothing but reject you
Is an act of
Revolution.
Be proud of a body
That bares the burden
Of being buried
Only to bloom.

Child,
How silly it is
That you cannot
See
Feel
Know
This vessel
Has carried you
Through your
Worst times,
And will carry you to
Your best
Minutes,
Moments,
Memories.
When your fingers
Brush your body
They are whispering
Thank you.

It's been a few months
Since the last time I cried.
My wells have run dry
But not because I miss you any less;
I finally accept that
This is life.
I can scream into
Every passing storm cloud,
But that will never bring you back.
I can yell at God
As I sob over crinkled pictures
But all I can grasp are memories.
There are days
I want to pretend
You are just a call away.
There are days I forget
Not only has your number
Been reassigned to a fast food joint,
There are days I forget
What your voice even sounded like.
But today is different.
This is life.
So I choose to remember your nails
Tracing up and down my back,
All the lessons you wove
Into your melodies,

Singing T Swift off-key.
I remind myself
(Because as much as we try,
It's too easy to forget)
That my God does not hate
Nor do They take.
You were not ripped away.
You floated away
In the arms of forgiveness,
And someday we will
Drift into the same inlet
And I will tell you
All the wonderful things
You have missed.

There's such adventure
In coffee swirls on our couch.
There's a whole world
Inside our pillow forts.
There is excitement
In cats leaping on our heads
In the middle of the movie.
There's laughter in
Cleaning up coffee
And popcorn spills.
There's a whole family,
Full
Furry
Finally happy.

Just as the chill seeps through
Our battered backdoor
And the cracks in my heart,
We will brave the winds
To bring home some warmth
About 6 feet tall.
These days getting shorter,
Our hugs getting longer;
Nights stringing lights
Remind me we're right.
This is the same feeling
As our very first year
When you and your parents
Put together my present.
We spent so much of that weekend
Tangled up in our stockings;
Putting up our tree,
You smile at me and
I'm glad to see
Even with the world
And the weather
Ever-changing,
You've got me
And you'll never leave.

I have 200 million
Reasons to keep going.

- You matter more than you know

Lost in my own brainwaves,
I have been swimming through
Tumultuous ocean waves
Since I could tread water.
I see myself,
Younger
Smaller,
Still my mother's daughter.
I see the currents
Threatening to pull me under
The weight of this trauma
On my shoulders.
I thank God I am older;
Reaching out,
I clutch onto myself.
Through these written words
I reach across time
And pull my soul
Through the riptides
That have ruled my life.
As these waters
Inevitably grow darker,
Time will bend
To the will of my pen;
Words remind me
I have survived tsunamis

In this lifetime,
And I have decades
Before I let this story
Float away from me.

Maybe we are

Never

Done healing.

Battle Armor

Gentle fingers rub
Oils and balms
Into my tender stomach,
Warm from my heat wrap.
All the things
This body overcomes
Bring a small smile
To my lips.
My body is fighting
This disease,
Not me.

Thank You

I lie with my feet
Propped up against
The wall;
You are playing
My favorite music
Through your Airpods
While vacuuming
And rearranging
Furniture.
The only help
I can offer
Is moving blankets
And making conversation.
That's enough.
I want to apologize
But I push a "thank you"
From my lips.
Thank you
For loving me
Even when I am bleeding.

Endo Fact Sheet

This is by no means the be-all-end-all of Endometriosis information, but this is a good place to start. I first and foremost want to say that if you are experiencing Endometriosis, I am incredibly proud of you every single day. On my lowest days, thinking of this community and talking to others who also have this disease has helped me beyond belief.

I want to let you know that no matter how you choose to treat your Endometriosis or its symptoms, you deserve relief. While I want you to be informed about every treatment or method of management, I don't want you to ever feel shame for the choices you have made or make. You're surviving, and that's incredible.

The last thing I will say in this preface is that Endometriosis - or Endo - is a very complex illness. Unfortunately, most OBGYNs are misinformed (for a multitude of reasons). Definitely, do your best to fact-check anything you see, talk to your qualified medical professional (which I am not), and continue to do your best! Now onto facts about Endometriosis.

- ○ Endometriosis is not the Endometrium! While Endometriosis is similar to the endometrium (the lining of the uterus), it is histologically and pathologically different. Endometriosis has been found in every organ of the body and is theorized to be implanted during our formation as fetuses. Basically, Endometriosis has been found in fetuses and infants but it often becomes worse with puberty and age.

○ The symptoms of Endometriosis include, but are not limited to:
  ○ Debilitating period pain
  ○ Pelvic and other (often abdominal) pain throughout the month
  ○ Leg pain most often associated with menstruation
  ○ Heavy or lengthy periods
  ○ Short or irregular periods
  ○ Periods that started before the age of 12
  ○ Bowel or urinary pain
  ○ Pain with intercourse and deep pain with penetration
  ○ Infertility or pregnancy loss
  ○ Any single or combination of allergies, autoimmune illness, chronic fatigue, chronic pain, and migraines may be associated with Endometriosis

It is important to note that not all people with Endometriosis will have these symptoms or comorbidities. The staging system is also very flawed and does not correlate with symptoms. This means that someone with Stage 1 disease may be in crippling pain, potentially all month long, while someone with Stage 4 disease might have no pain but be experiencing infertility. Each person's experience with Endometriosis is very different, and so many of the symptoms vary and can also change over time. If you feel you are experiencing these symptoms, it is important to record your symptoms and bring them up with your doctor. You know more about your body than anyone else in this world; trust your instincts.

○   Endometriosis also does not follow the same patterns as the endometrium, which is why we can have pain at any point in our cycles.

○   There is no cure!

○   There is only one true treatment for Endometriosis, excision surgery. Excision surgery with an Endometriosis specialist is the gold standard of care, but it is widely inaccessible to most patients. There are other surgeries performed for Endometriosis, though none of them are proven to be as effective as excision; these include ablation, diagnostic, and hysterectomy.

○   An important note is that **a hysterectomy does not help Endometriosis.** It is a cure for Adenomyosis, which many Endo patients have, and explains why some do get relief from a hysterectomy. Ablation only burns the top of Endometriosis lesions, often leaving behind some of the painful disease. For these reasons, excision is considered the gold standard of care. Unfortunately, it is much more costly and there are few qualified surgeons, so many patients are not able to access this care.

○   Similarly, there are no medications that "treat" Endometriosis. There are some medications that may help you manage your symptoms, but not always. Some doctors recommend birth control, progesterone, or even Lupron or Orilissa. It is important to note that none of these medications actually treats Endometriosis. Some people experience relief on these medications, but they do not treat Endometriosis. The Endometriosis does still grow while on these medications but your symptoms might be managed. Some of these medications are also safer than others. There are many long-term side effects associated with Lupron and Orilissa, and they were both approved by the FDA using falsified data. Lupron and Orilissa continue to advertise false data to patients, so please do your research and decide what path is best for you. However you choose to manage your disease, I truly hope you are able to find relief.

○   The only true way to diagnose Endometriosis is through laparoscopic surgery. A surgeon will go in through a small hole in the belly button and look for the Endo and should send anything they find for a pathology report. Unfortunately, many surgeons are not trained in how to find all forms of Endometriosis, so a negative laparoscopy does not always mean you do not have Endometriosis. Similarly, if you have not been able to or do not want a laparoscopy, that is valid. Your symptoms and diagnosis are still valid and you still belong in this community. Remember, you know more about your body than anyone else in this world; trust your instincts.

○   You are incredibly strong! Endometriosis was listed as one of the top 20 most painful conditions one can experience. It is said to be as painful or more painful than labor, kidney stones, and heart attacks. Don't let anyone tell you the pain is all in your head; you are fighting an incredibly painful whole-body disease. I am proud of you!

Endometriosis Resouces

Sources to reference (note: I do not agree with some of the political affiliations of some of the employees/doctors, but their websites do have lots of factual and up to date research and information about Endometriosis):

- ○ Center for Endometriosis Care, Atlanta, GA
- ○ Endopaedia.info
- ○ Nancysnookendo.com
- ○ endo.icarebetter.com
- ○ The podcast and website insixteenyears.com

Friendos on Instagram:

- ○ in16yearsofendo
- ○ mypelvicpain
- ○ me_myself_and_endometriosis
- ○ endogram
- ○ endohealthhub
- ○ theendojournal
- ○ beelynnnyc

Other Books:

- Vagina Problems by Lara Parker
- Finding Peace with a Devastating Disease: Reflections on Endometriosis by Amy Corfeli
- Know Your Endo by Jessica Murnane
- Beating Endo by Iris Orbuch and Amy Stein
- Ask Me About My Uterus by Abby Norman
- Living with Endometriosis by Samantha Bowick
- How to Endo by Bridget Hustwaite
- Private Parts by Eleanor Thom
- The Doctor Will See You Now by Tamer Seckin

"I want my friendos to feel seen and understood. I want to reach out through a book in the middle of your flare and hold you, hold space for you. And I want you to be able to give this to your loved ones and say 'see me, please.'" - Maggie Bowyer

Maggie Bowyer (they/them/theirs) is a poet and the author of *The Whole Story* (Margaret Bowyer, 2020) and *When I Bleed* (Margaret Bowyer, 2021). They are a blogger and essayist with a focus on Endometriosis and chronic pain. They have been featured in Detour Ahead, Germ Magazine, Scribe, A Cornered Gurl, Written Tales, P.S. I Love You, Scholastic, The People's Poetry Podcast, Teen Ink, Poetry 365, and more. They were the Editor-in-Chief of The Lariat Newspaper, a semi-finalist in Brave New Voices 2016, and were a Marilyn Miller Poet Laureate.

CPSIA information can be obtained
at www.ICGtesting.com
Printed in the USA
BVHW042343230421
605782BV00004B/25